Body Butter Recipes

By
Gene Ashburner

ISBN-13:978-1508459828
ISBN-10:1508459827

Contents

Body Butter

Body butter is excellent for very dry skin especially on elbows, feet and knees. It smoothes and softens the skin.

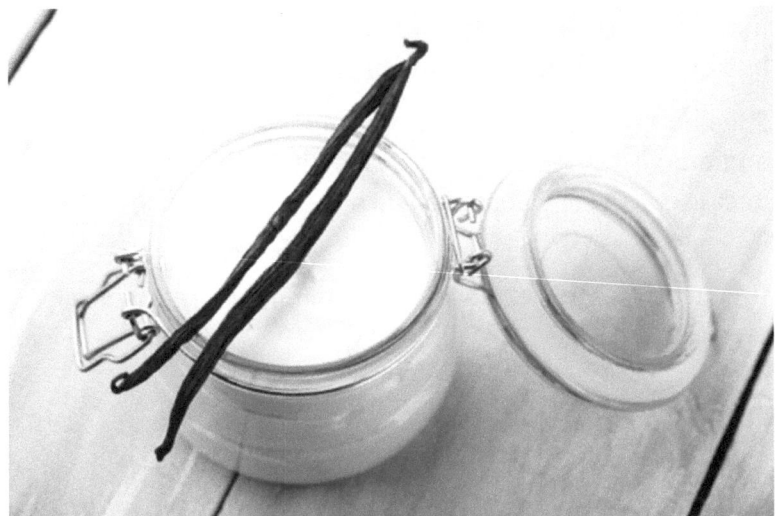

Common Ingredients Used In Body Butter

Shea Butter

Shea butter is also known as shea nut butter. It is a naturally-occurring fat found in the fruit of shea trees. The butter is extracted by means of crushing or boiling.

Shea butter has a reputation for being a good moisturizer and emollient because it contains Vitamins A, E and F and because it's easily absorbed into the skin while softening it.

Unlike other fats, it doesn't leave behind a greasy or oily residue.

Apricot Kernel Oil

Vitamins A and B help in healing and rejuvenating skin cells.

It contains vitamin E.

Cocoa Butter

Cocoa butter is a pure edible vegetable fat extracted from the cocoa bean. It is the most stable known fat. The stable fat, together with natural antioxidants grant it a shelf life of 2 to 5 years.

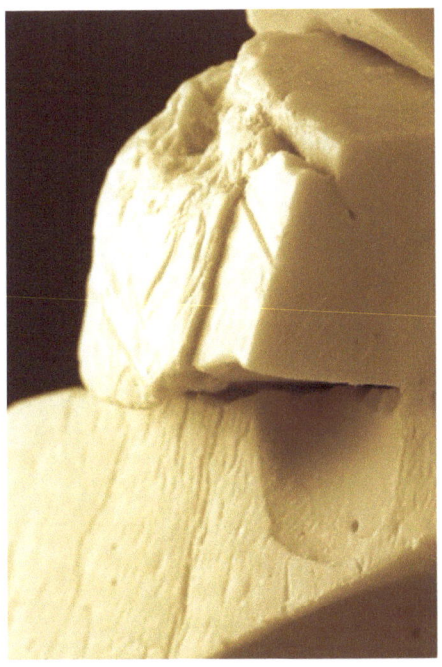

The velvety texture, fragrance and emollient properties of cocoa butter have made it a popular ingredient for cosmetics, soaps and lotions.

The moisturizing abilities of cocoa butter are recommended for the treatment of chapped skin and lips and as a daily moisturizer to prevent dry, itchy skin.

Essential Oils

Essential oils are the concentrated essence of plant material widely used in aromatherapy. They are exclusively made from botanical matter.

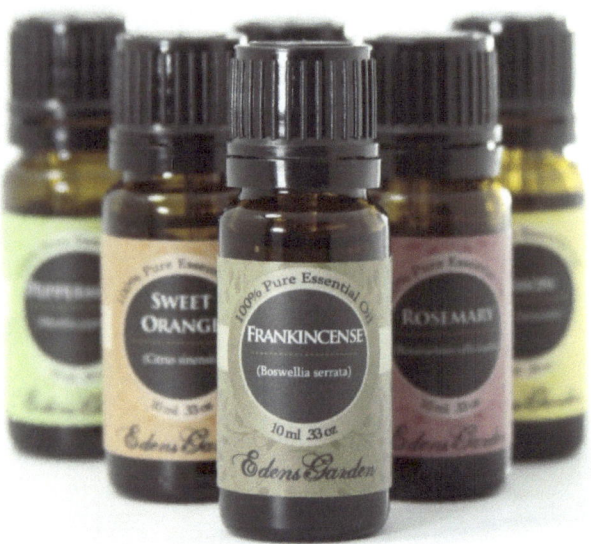

Sweet Almond Oil

This oil Provides relief from itching, soreness, dryness, inflammation.

Beeswax

Beeswax is a natural wax produced in the bee hive of honey bees. A German study found beeswax to be superior to similar "barrier creams" such as mineral oil based creams.

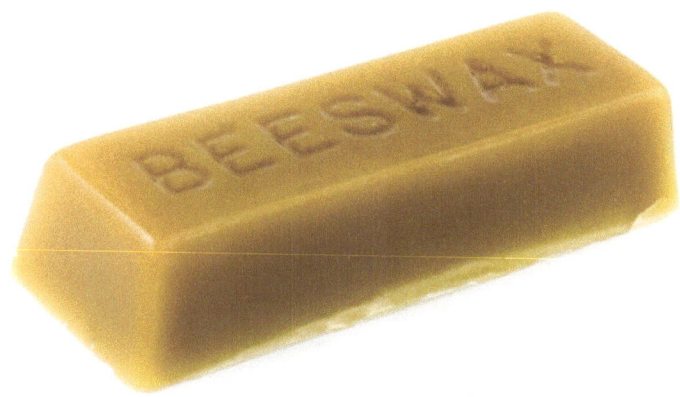

Wheat Germ Oil

A highly nourishing oil with vitamin E.

Jojoba Oil

It heals inflamed skin, psoriasis, eczema, or any sort of dermatitis.

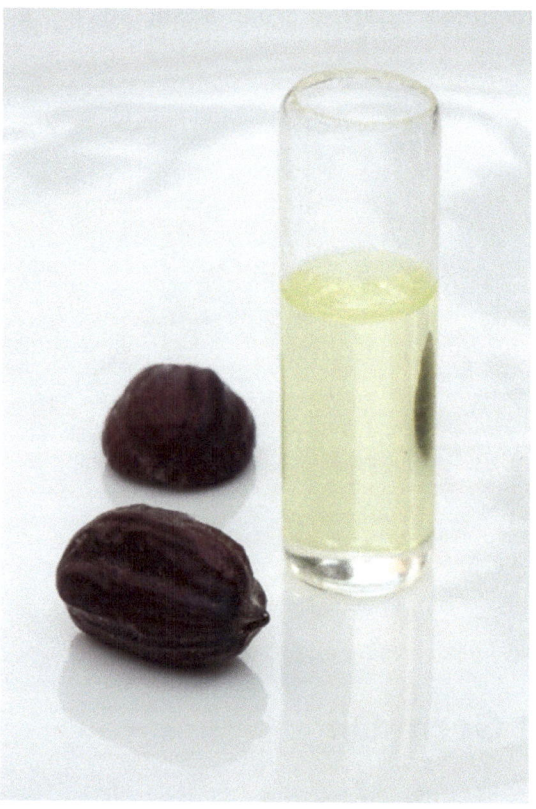

Rose Hip Oil

Good oil for cosmetic, cell regeneration prevents premature skin aging and softens wrinkles.

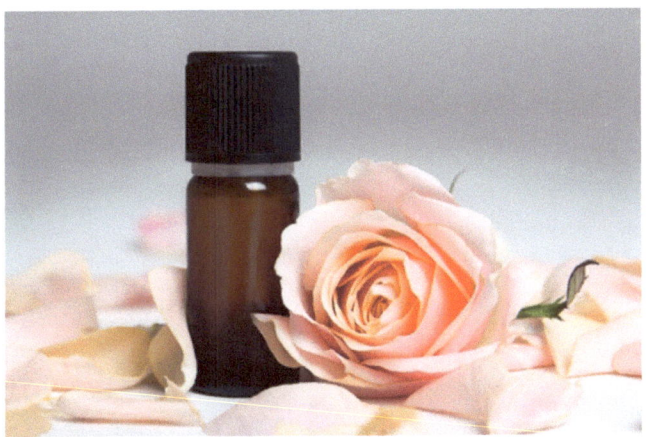

Evening Primrose Oil

Perfect skincare oil for moisturizing, softening and soothing to dry and irritated skin.

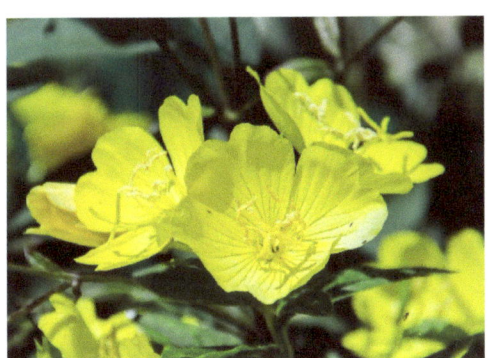

Evening Primrose Flowers

Recipes

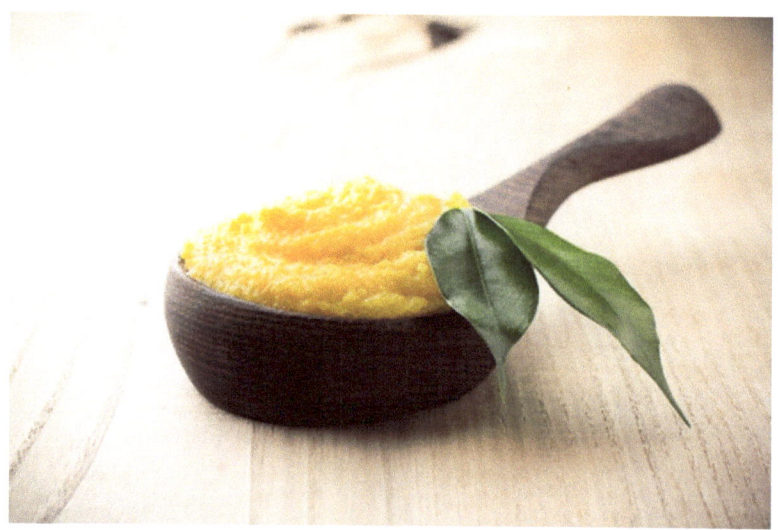

Almond Body Butter

Ingredients

375 ml shea butter

187 ml cocoa butter

187 ml sweet almond oil

125 ml ground almonds

Method

Combine the shea butter and cocoa butter together in a double boiler.

Stir and melt the ingredients.

Remove the mixture from the heat.

Leave the mixture to cool.

Add the sweet almond oil and ground almonds.

Whisk the mixture with an electric hand beater.

Freeze the mixture for 5 minutes.

Whisk the mixture for 5 minutes with the electric beater.

Freeze the mixture for 5 minutes.

Whisk the mixture for 5 minutes with the electric beater.

Continue this process until the body butter form peaks.

Store the body butter in a glass jar with a lid.

Apricot Body Butter

Ingredients

375 ml shea butter

187 ml cocoa butter

187 ml apricot kernel oil

Method

Combine the shea butter and cocoa butter together in a double boiler.

Stir and melt the ingredients.

Remove the mixture from the heat.

Leave the mixture to cool.

Add the apricot kernel oil.

Whisk the mixture with an electric hand beater.

Freeze the mixture for 5 minutes.

Whisk the mixture for 5 minutes with the electric beater.

Freeze the mixture for 5 minutes.

Whisk the mixture for 5 minutes with the electric beater.

Continue this process until the body butter form peaks.

Store the body butter in a glass jar with a lid.

Avocado Body Butter

Ingredients

250 ml cocoa butter (grated)

50ml beeswax (grated)

50 ml grape seed oil

50 ml avocado (mashed)

Method

Combine the cocoa butter and beeswax together in a double boiler.

Melt the mixture.

Remove the mixture from the heat.

Beat in the grape seed oil and avocado.

Mix well.

Leave for 10 minutes.

Whisk again.

Store the body butter in a jar with a lid.

Beeswax Almond Oil Body Butter

Ingredients

200 ml beeswax

200 ml cocoa butter

200 ml almond oil

Method

Melt the beeswax and cocoa butter together in a double boiler.

Add the almond oil.

Mix very well.

Store the body butter in a jar with a lid.

Beeswax Apricot Body Butter

Ingredients

1250 ml apricot kernel oil

250 ml cocoa butter

250 ml beeswax

Method

Melt the apricot kernel oil, cocoa butter and beeswax in a double boiler.

Beat with a wooden spoon until the body butter is smooth and cooled.

Store the body butter in a jar with a lid.

Beeswax Coconut Body Butter

Ingredients

250 ml beeswax

150 ml baby oil

250 ml coconut oil

343 ml glycerine

Method

Combine the beeswax and coconut oil together in a double boiler.

Stir until the mixture has melted.

Add the baby oil and glycerine.

Heat until the mixture is smooth.

Pour into a jar with a lid.

Beeswax Mango Body Butter

Ingredients

250 ml beeswax

250 ml coconut oil

250 ml apricot kernel oil

5 ml essential oil of choice

62,5 ml mango butter

Method

Melt all the ingredients together in a double boiler.

Mix well until the body butter is smooth.

Pour into a jar with a lid.

Butter Lotion Bars

Ingredients

4 oz cocoa butter

4 oz beeswax

4 oz shea butter

Method

Melt the cocoa butter, beeswax and shea butter together in a double boiler.

Mix very well.

Pour the melted mixture into a mold.

Evening Primrose Body Butter

Ingredients

375 ml shea butter

187 ml cocoa butter

187 ml evening primrose oil

Method

Combine the shea butter and cocoa butter together in a double boiler.

Stir and melt the ingredients.

Remove the mixture from the heat.

Leave the mixture to cool.

Add the evening primrose oil.

Whisk the mixture with an electric hand beater.

Freeze the mixture for 5 minutes.

Whisk the mixture for 5 minutes with the electric beater.

Freeze the mixture for 5 minutes.

Whisk the mixture for 5 minutes with the electric beater.

Continue this process until the body butter form peaks.

Store the body butter in a glass jar with a lid.

Grape Seed And Citrus Body Butter

Ingredients

50 ml beeswax

250 ml grape seed oil

2 capsules vitamin E oil

75 ml distilled water

20 drops citrus essential oil

Method

Combine the beeswax, grape seed oil and vitamin E oil together.

Microwave until the mixture until it is almost completely melted.

Whip the mixture with a hand blender.

Slowly add the water.

Continue to whip mixture.

Add the citrus essential oil.

Mix well.

Leave the mixture for 20 minutes.

Scoop the body butter into a container and seal.

Honey Beeswax Body Butter

Ingredients

250 ml beeswax

250 ml petroleum jelly

250 ml almond oil

250 ml honey

50 ml bee pollen

250 ml glycerin

50 ml liquid lecithin

Method

Melt the beeswax and petroleum jelly together in double boiler.

Add the almond oil, honey, bee pollen, glycerine and liquid lecithin.

Mix well and heat for 5 minutes.

Mix until smooth.

Scoop the body butter into a container and seal.

Jojoba And Aloe Vera Body Butter

Ingredients

50 g jojoba oil

20 g beeswax

20 g cocoa butter

25 ml vitamin E oil

100 g Aloe Vera

20 g glycerine

60 drops essential oil of choice

Method

Combine the jojoba, beeswax, cocoa butter and vitamin E together in a double boiler.

Heat to 160 degrees F.

Combine the Aloe Vera and glycerine together in a double boiler.

Heat to 160 degrees F.

Combine the 2 mixtures slowly, stir continuously.

Stir until the mixture cools to 80 degrees F.

Add the essential oils.

Mix well.

Pour the body butter into a jar with a lid.

Mint Body Butter

Ingredients

20 oz shea butter

6 oz sunflower oil

6 oz coconut oil

20 ml corn starch

2 oz peppermint oil

Method

Melt the shea butter in a double boiler.

When the shea butter has melted, add the sunflower oil, coconut oil, peppermint oil and corn starch.

Blend very well.

Remove the mixture from the heat.

Place the bowl containing the mixture into a bowl filled with ice water for a cold water bath.

This will help cool the body butter faster.

Whip the butter continually for several minutes with an electric beater.

Once the butter has solidified and forms peaks it is ready.

Spoon the body butter into jars.

Orange Almond Body Butter

Ingredients

20 oz shea butter

6 oz almond oil

6 oz coconut oil

20 ml corn starch

2 oz orange oil

Method

Melt the shea butter in a double boiler.

When the shea butter has melted, add the almond oil, coconut oil, orange oil and corn starch.

Blend very well.

Remove the mixture from the heat.

Place the bowl containing the mixture into a bowl filled with ice water for a cold water bath.

This will help cool the body butter faster.

Whip the butter continually for several minutes with an electric beater.

Once the butter has solidified and forms peaks it is ready.

Spoon the body butter into jars.

Rosehip Oil Body Butter

Ingredients

375 ml shea butter

187 ml cocoa butter

187 ml rose hip oil

Method

Combine the shea butter and cocoa butter together in a double boiler.

Stir and melt the ingredients.

Remove the mixture from the heat.

Leave the mixture to cool.

Add the rose hip oil.

Whisk the mixture with an electric hand beater.

Freeze the mixture for 5 minutes.

Whisk the mixture for 5 minutes with the electric beater.

Freeze the mixture for 5 minutes.

Whisk the mixture for 5 minutes with the electric beater.

Continue this process until the body butter form peaks.

Store the body butter in a glass jar with a lid.

Shea Body Butter

Ingredients

375 ml shea butter

187 ml cocoa butter

187 ml jojoba oil

Method

Combine the shea butter and cocoa butter together in a double boiler.

Stir and melt the ingredients.

Remove the mixture from the heat.

Leave the mixture to cool.

Add the jojoba oil.

Whisk the mixture with an electric hand beater.

Freeze the mixture for 5 minutes.

Whisk the mixture for 5 minutes with the electric beater.

Freeze the mixture for 5 minutes.

Whisk the mixture for 5 minutes with the electric beater.

Continue this process until the body butter form peaks.

Store the body butter in a glass jar with a lid.

Wheat Germ Body Butter

Ingredients

375 ml shea butter

187 ml cocoa butter

187 ml wheat germ oil

Method

Combine the shea butter and cocoa butter together in a double boiler.

Stir and melt the ingredients.

Remove the mixture from the heat.

Leave the mixture to cool.

Add the wheat germ oil.

Whisk the mixture with an electric hand beater.

Freeze the mixture for 5 minutes.

Whisk the mixture for 5 minutes with the electric beater.

Freeze the mixture for 5 minutes.

Whisk the mixture for 5 minutes with the electric beater.

Continue this process until the body butter form peaks.

Store the body butter in a glass jar with a lid.